Modified Keto Diet

A 3-Week Step-by-Step Guide for Beginners, with Curated Recipes and a Sample Meal Plan

LARRY JAMESONN

Introduction

According to statistics, 36.5% of American adults are obese. More specifically, 40% (aged 40–59) are likely obese, and a third (aged 60 and above) are diagnosed obese.

For younger individuals aged 20–39, around 32.3% of them are obese. Whereas children between the ages of 2 to 19, around 17% are overweight. This poses a risk because overweight children tend to grow up obese.

Sadly, obesity is a problem not limited to America. Obesity is found in the top five leading causes of death. According to the World Health Organization (WHO), obesity causes 2.8 million fatalities around the world every year. More and more people are becoming overweight. The increase in the obesity rate all over the world is attributed to poor diet and unhealthy eating choices.

In America alone, studies claim that Americans are consuming more calories now than ever.

An unhealthy diet that is linked to obesity is composed of refined sugars, trans fats, sodium, and excess calories. A diet loaded with rice, bread, potatoes, fruit juices, sugar, and pasta lead to an increased risk of health issues related to the liver, heart, brain, gut, and pancreas.

Fortunately, obesity is preventable and one of the methods that you can follow is the Modified Keto Diet, which helps you achieve your ideal weight and health goals.

This guide that you now hold aims to:

- Educate you about the proper approach to dieting
- Introduce you to a better form of keto
- Help you make the right food choices
- Make your diet easier
- Teach you how to make healthy food

Table of Contents

A FUN WAY TO KETO

Traditional Keto

The ketogenic diet entered the limelight when celebrities started popularizing it. It was initially developed as a diet plan for epilepsy and is now a lifestyle of its own. It is a low-carb, high-fat diet with a macronutrient ratio of 70-75% fat, 5-10% carbohydrates, and 20-25% protein. This means that 5 – 10 % of a 2,000-calorie diet is equal to 50 grams of carbs daily.

The human body creates fuel by breaking down carbohydrates through a biochemical process called glycolysis.

Once your carbohydrate storage is used up, your body looks for an alternative, eventually metabolizing your stored fats to generate energy—this is called ketosis.

The idea behind this is that, in a keto diet, you limit your carbohydrate intake so that you can burn your untouched fats. By doing so, you can use up your fat storage faster and eventually lose weight.

Ketosis is a natural biochemical process that our bodies go through to come up with fuel when there are no carbohydrates available or when we are in a fasting state.

Based on studies, it can trigger weight loss, and manage epilepsy and type 2 diabetes.

Despite its promising effects, its strict limitations make it difficult to sustain. Some experience a temporary phase at the beginning called the "keto flu," where they complain of fatigue, headache, nausea, foggy brain, constipation, difficulty sleeping, and irritability. However, these symptoms usually go away once the body has acclimated to the new diet.

Another concern is that it is easy to develop micronutrient deficiencies because of its restrictive nature. Since you need to allow up to 75% of your daily caloric intake to be fat, this leaves little room for anything else. By following the keto diet, you tend to lack nutrients commonly found in starchy fruits and vegetables. The most common nutrients lacking are folate, fiber, magnesium, vitamin C, calcium, and magnesium. The lack of fiber also leads to constipation and indigestion. Research on the long-term benefits of the keto diet is lacking. This is why dietitians only recommend the keto diet to be implemented for 3–12 months.

What is the Modified Keto Diet?

Simply put, the modified keto diet is the less restrictive and more laid-back version of the keto diet. Most beginners in the keto diet are unknowingly following a modified keto diet. In the modified keto diet, around 50–60% of your diet is still fat, 25–30% of protein, and 15–20% of carbohydrates. Keep in mind though that by raising your carbohydrate intake to 20%, your body might not reach ketosis at all.

Benefits of Modified Keto Diet

1. Modified Keto allows for more fiber.

One of the side effects of the traditional keto diet is constipation. The traditional keto diet only allows 5–10 % of carbs which restricts the consumption of starchy carbohydrates that contain fiber. Fiber is necessary for digestion. In the modified keto diet, the increase in the daily carbohydrate intake allows us to incorporate more starchy carbohydrates and dietary fiber into our diets.

2. Modified Keto is better for the muscle.

People swear that they lose weight on the keto diet. But the truth is they are not only shedding excess fat, but they could also be shedding their lean muscles too. According to nutritionists, consuming 75% of fat and 20% protein daily in the keto diet could lead to muscle loss. The increase in protein intake helps to maintain the lean muscle mass of the body.

3. Modified Keto diet promotes the consumption of healthy fats.

People on a high-fat diet tend to eat anything fatty just to reach their daily macro quota. This could lead to higher cholesterol levels and increase the risk of heart problems. In the modified keto diet, the daily fat requirement needs to come from healthy fats.

4. The modified Keto diet is more nutrient-dense.

One of the main drawbacks of the traditional keto diet is nutrient deficiency. The new macronutrient ratio of the modified keto diet allows more wiggle room to include nutrient-rich foods in our daily diet.

5. The modified Keto diet is easier to follow.

The traditional keto diet is very restrictive and challenging to follow especially for children. Modifying the ratio of the macronutrients makes it easier for children in therapy to adhere to the diet. It is also a great starting point or transition phase for beginners in the keto diet. The modified keto diet also lessens the side effects brought by the traditional keto diet.

DIET AND EXERCISE

Can I still lose weight in the Modified Keto Diet?

Most dietitians agree that weight loss is possible in the Modified Keto Diet. If done correctly, a modified keto diet still promotes weight loss albeit slower than the traditional keto diet. Since ketosis is not achieved in the modified keto diet, weight loss happens gradually. The results are more evident in people with unhealthy lifestyles and diets before trying the modified keto diet. The best way to go about this is to set short-term and long-term goals. Your short-term goals could include losing 1 kilo every week or 10 lbs. every month. This way you can monitor your progress.

Modified Keto Diet and HIIT exercises

Following a Modified Keto diet alone, already guarantees weight loss. But most health experts agree that a healthy life is not dependent on diet alone. Being proactive also helps our overall health and disposition. Here is some easy, no-equipment HIIT exercise you could do:

1. Butt Kicks

Start by jogging in place. While jogging, make sure that your ankles reach your butt.

2. Air Punches

Stand straight, hip-width apart. Punch each arm alternately in front of you.

3. High Knees

Think of this as the opposite of Butt kicks. Stand straight and bend your elbows 90 degrees to the front with your palms facing down. Jog on spot making sure that your knees touch your palms.

4. Mountain Climbers

Start in a high plank position with your hands beneath your shoulders. In this position, move your feet as if you're climbing. Do this without rocking your torso side to side.

5. Walkout

Start by standing straight. Slide your hands downward until it reaches the floor. Crawl down until you reach a high plank position. Stay in the plank for a few seconds then walk your hand back to the standing position.

6. Star jump

Stand up with feet hip-width apart. Go down in squat form and touch your toes. From this position, jump upward while extending your arms.

7. Downward Dog Toe Tap

Start in a downward dog position. Lift your left hand and touch your right toe. Return to the downward dog position. Repeat with the other hand.

KNOW YOUR MACROS

Understanding Macronutrients

For any diet to succeed, understanding macronutrients are essential. Most people assume that just because they are cutting down one macro means they don't need to put importance on the other two. Some individuals chug down on unhealthy choices just to amp the macro that they need to consume more. This is the reason why most diets don't work.

1.Carbohydrates are the body's primary fuel source. Our body uses carbohydrates by default because it is easier to convert and readily available. Glycolysis is the process of breaking down carbohydrates into glucose. Carbohydrates are needed by our muscles, cells, and our brain to function. Carbohydrates contain 4 kcal per gram.

There are two types of carbohydrates:

A. Complex carbohydrates – are long strings of sugar called polysaccharides or oligosaccharides. Complex carbohydrates provide our body with a steadier source of energy and keep our blood glucose levels. Common sources include starchy vegetables, pasta, bread, grains, nuts, and rice. Complex carbohydrates also contain dietary fiber which is necessary for healthy digestive function. dietitians recommend consuming more complex carbohydrates than simple carbohydrates.

B. Simple Carbohydrates – are carbohydrates that usually contain one or two strings of sugar. They provide our body with short bursts of energy and have a fleeting impact on our blood glucose levels. Common sources include table sugar, honey, maple, molasses, syrup, and fruits.

2. Protein plays an important role in maintaining, repairing, and protecting our bodies. Protein is made up of amino acids. We can produce 11 types of amino acids in our bodies. However, there are 9 types of amino acids that our body needs but can't produce. These are called essential amino acids. Dietitians recommend a daily intake of 10 – 35% of protein. Protein contains 4 kcal per gram.

There are two types of protein:

A. Complete protein – provides all the needed amino acids in sufficient amounts. Common sources include seafood, poultry, meat, eggs, and milk.

B. Incomplete protein – provides some of the essential amino acids or in insufficient amounts. Most plant-based protein sources are incomplete proteins. Sources include nuts, most grains, and seeds.

3. Fat is essential in proper cell function, and organ insulation and protection. It also helps in vitamin absorption, body temperature maintenance, and hormone production. In times of caloric deprivation, our body burns down stored fats

into ketones to fuel our body. Studies claim that ketones are a much more efficient source of energy for our bodies. Fat contains 9 kcal per gram.

There are two types of fat:

A. Saturated fats - are generally solid at room temperature and have a longer shelf life. Past studies claim that high consumption of saturated fats leads to high cholesterol levels and increases the risk of heart diseases. Common sources include cheese, butter, fatty meats, lard, and lamb.

B. Unsaturated fats – are usually in liquid form at room temperature and shorter shelf life. Unlike saturated fats, unsaturated fats are good for the heart as it lessens the risk of heart disease. This is why unsaturated fats are dubbed healthy fats. Common sources include plant-based oils, seeds and nuts, seed butter and nut butter, avocados, olives, and fatty fish like herring, sardines, tuna, and mackerel.

WHAT'S IN MY PLATE?

The following may be used as a guide or basis to check the protein, fat, and carbohydrate contents per serving equivalent to specific serving sizes.

Protein Content of Foods

Food (cooked)	Serving Size	Calories per serving	Protein (g) per serving
Lobster	3 oz.	76	16
Salmon	3 oz.	155	22
Scallops	3 oz.	75	14
Shrimp	3 oz.	101	20
Tuna	3 oz.	99	22
Adzuki Beans	1/2 cup	147	9
Black Beans	1/2 cup	114	8
Black-eyed Peas	1/2 cup	100	7
Chickpeas	1/2 cup	134	7
Edamame	1/2 cup	95	9
Fava Beans	1/2 cup	94	7
Green Peas	1/2 cup	59	4
Kamut	1/2 cup	126	6
Lima Beans	1/2 cup	105	6
Pinto Beans	1/2 cup	197	11
Quinoa	1/2 cup	111	4
Red Kidney Beans	1/2 cup	112	8
Spinach	1/2 cup	41	3
Wheat Beans	1/2 cup	151	6
Almonds	1 oz.	163	6
Cashews	1 oz.	162	4
Chia seeds	1 oz.	138	5
Flax seeds	1 oz.	140	6
Peanuts	1 oz.	166	7

Food (cooked)	Serving Size	Calories per serving	Protein (g) per serving
Peanut Butter	1 tbsp	188	7
Pumpkin Seeds	1 oz.	159	9
Pistachios	1 oz.	161	6
Soy nuts	1 oz.	120	12
Sunflower seeds	1 oz.	140	6
Walnuts	1 oz.	185	4
Chicken, skinless	3 oz.	141	28
Egg, large	1 piece	71	6
Ham	3 oz.	139	14
Lamb	3 oz.	172	23
Pork	3 oz.	122	22
Steak	3 oz.	158	26
Roasted turkey	3 oz.	135	25
Cottage Cheese	4 oz.	81	14
Greek Yogurt	6 oz.	100	18
Milk	1 cup	86	8
Mozzarella	1 oz.	72	7
Soy Milk	1 cup	132	8
String cheese	.75 oz.	50	6
Yogurt	1 cup	100	11
Yellow corn	1 cup	59	15.6
Broccoli	1 cup	31	3
Brussels sprouts	½ cup	28	2
Cauliflower	1 cup	27	2

Carbohydrate Content of Foods

Food	Serving Size	Calories per serving	Carbohydrates per serving (g)
Apple	1 medium	21	81
Banana	1 piece	27	105
Cantaloupe	1 cup	14	57
Dried Dates	10 pieces	61	228
Grapes	1 cup	28	114
Orange	1 piece	16	65
Pear	1 piece	25	98
Pineapple	1 cup	19	77
Dried Prunes	10 pieces	53	201
Raspberries	1 cup	14	61
Strawberries	1 cup	11	45
Watermelon	1 cup	12	50
Black-eyed peas	1/2 cup	22	134
Carrot	1 medium	8	31
Corn	1/2 cup	21	89
Chickpeas	1 cup	45	269
Lima beans (cooked)	1/2 cup	20	108
Green Peas	1/2 cup	12	63
Navy beans	1 cup	48	259
Pinto Beans	1 cup	44	235
Potato (plain baked)	1 large	50	220
Sweet potato	1 large	28	118
White beans	1 cup	45	249
Chocolate milk	1 cup	26	208
Pudding	1/2 cup	30	161
Skim milk	1 cup	12	86
Apple juice	1 cup	28	111
Grape juice	1 cup	28	114
Orange juice	1 cup	26	112

Food	Serving Size	Calories per serving	Carbohydrates per serving (g)
Bagel	1 piece	31	165
Biscuit	1 piece	13	103
Breadsticks	2 pieces	15	77
Bread, white	1 slice	12	61
Bread, whole wheat	1 slice	11	55
Cereal	1 cup	24	110
Oatmeal raisin cookie	1 piece	9	62
Cornbread	1 piece	28	178
English Muffin	1 piece	25	130
Fig bar	1 piece	10	50
Graham crackers	2 squares	11	60
Honey and oats granola bar	1 oz.	19	125
Bun, hamburger	1 piece	21	119
Bun, hotdog	1 piece	21	119
Spaghetti noodles	1 cup	12	66
Instant oatmeal	1 packet	25	110
Oatmeal	1/2 cup	12	66
Cheese pizza	1 slice	39	290
Popcorn, plain popped	1 cup	6	26
Pretzels	1 oz.	21	106
Rice, white	1 cup	50	223
Rice, brown	1 cup	50	232
Saltine crackers	5 pieces	10	60
Tortilla (flour)	1 piece	15	85

Fat Content of Foods

Food	Serving Size	Fat per serving (Grams)	Other benefits
Avocado	1 piece	21	9 g of fiber
Walnuts	1 oz.	21	Rich in omega-3 and omega-6 fatty acids, copper, and manganese
Almonds	1 oz.	15	Rich in vitamin E
Peanut Butter	2 tbsp	16	Rich in fiber and protein
Olives	1 oz.	4	
Olive oil	1 tbsp	14	
Ground flaxseed		8	Rich in fiber
Salmon	3 oz.	11	Source of omega-3 fatty acids
Tuna	1 can	5	Omega-3 fatty acids
Dark chocolate	1 oz.	11	fiber
Tofu	3 oz.	4	Plant-based source of protein
Edamame (shelled)	½ cup	4.5	9g. of protein and 4g. the fiber in 1 serving
Sunflower seeds	2 tbsp	14	6g. of protein and 2g. fiber per serving
Chia seeds	2 tbsp	6	Packed with essential minerals, fiber, protein, and healthy fats.
Eggs	1 whole large	6	Contains necessary minerals and vitamins, protein-rich
Hemp seeds	3 tbsp	15	9g. of protein per serving

Anchovies	2 oz.	4.5	Full of healthy fats and protein
Pumpkin seeds	1 oz.	13	Provides protein, magnesium, copper, manganese, iron, and phosphorus
Macadamia Nuts	1 oz.	22	Has adequate amounts of protein per serving
Cheese	1 slice		Calcium, phosphorous, selenium, vitamin b12, protein
Coconut oil	1 tbsp	7	

WEEK 1 MODIFIED KETO DIET SAMPLE MEAL PLAN

	AM (breakfast and snack)	Noon (lunch and snack)	PM (dinner and snack)
Day 1	Scrambled eggs	Tomato soup	Cucumber Salad
	Goats milk yogurt	Apple with almond butter	
Day 2	Mushroom Mini Frittatas	Cajun Parmesan Salmon	Slow Cooker French Onion Soup
	Macadamia nuts	Bacon-wrapped shrimp and scallops	
Day 3	Keto Banana Bread	Keto chili	Spicy Beef Ramen
	Seaweed snacks	Pork rinds	

Day			
Day 4	Bulletproof coffee and hard-boiled eggs	Salmon and Green Salad	Thai Beef Lettuce Wraps
	Bacon-wrapped shrimp and scallops	Kale chips	
Day 5	Chorizo Omelette	Cabbage Soup	Grilled salmon and spinach
	Celery and pepper strips	Crab and Avocado duet	
Day 6	Keto Naan bread	Curried Chicken Skillet	Turkey chili and vegetable salad
	Roast beef and sliced cheese	Sugar-free turkey jerky	
Day 7	Corned Beef and Cauliflower hash	Taco Salad	Stuffed Pork Roast
	Apple with almond butter	Bell Pepper Nachos	

FACING NUTRIENT DEFICIENCIES

Nutrient Deficiencies related to a Low Carbohydrate Diet and How to Remedy It

1. Folate or Vitamin B9

Vitamin B9 or folate is essential in methylation, a chemical process that enables our cells to function. Methylation also plays a role in gene expression, energy production, mood control, hormone balancing, and cravings. Folate controls the neurotransmitter that is responsible for our happiness, sense of contentment, and urges. Most low-carb dieters fail to limit their eating portions because of the lack of folate. Vitamin B9 is commonly found in whole foods, which typically have high carbohydrate content. Our body needs around 400 mcg of folate daily.

Remedy

- Low carb sources: leafy vegetables, avocado, chicken liver, salmon, and lamb.
- Try taking active folate supplements, which can be readily used by the body.

2. Thiamine

Thiamine or Vitamin B1 is important in nervous and brain functions, as well as energy production. Vitamin B1 works in conjunction with other B Vitamins. This means that a deficiency in one will affect the synthesis of the others. dietitians suggest a daily requirement of 1.1mg of thiamine.

Remedy

- Low carb sources: Asparagus, Pecans, chicken livers, flaxseed, pork loin, almonds

3. Calcium

This plays a major role in bone development and strength. It is also essential in balancing the acid and base of our body. Calcium is also needed by our nerves and muscles to function properly. RDA recommends a daily calcium intake of 1000mg.

Remedy

- Low carb sources: sardines, tofu, canned salmon, kale

4. Magnesium

For magnesium, this plays a supporting role in protein synthesis, DNA synthesis, bone maintenance and development, and cell function. It also helps in blood sugar control, prevents constipation, and aids in keeping the body calm during stressful moments. Women need around 310 mg of magnesium daily and 400mg for men.

Remedy

- Low carb sources: avocado, spinach, almonds, flaxseed, pumpkin seeds, soybeans

5. Potassium

Potassium is responsible for regulating the body's fluid levels and controlling muscle contractions. Potassium deficiency could lead to fatigue, constipation, and muscle weakness. In general, men need to take around 3000-3400 mg of potassium daily while women need 2300-2600 mg.

Remedy

- Low carb sources: mushrooms, avocado, spinach, green leafy vegetables.

6. Selenium

Selenium is a multiplayer mineral. It plays an essential role in maintaining heart health, encourages blood flow, and maintains normal thyroid functions and hormone production. Selenium is also an antioxidant that protects the body from free radicals. Although selenium deficiencies are rarely life-threatening, a high-fat diet is generally low in selenium.

Remedy

- Low carb sources: brazil nuts, shrimps, sardines, oysters, liver, tuna, and meat

Week 2 Modified Keto Diet Sample Meal Plan

	AM (breakfast and snack)	Noon (lunch and snack)	PM (dinner and snack)
Day 1	Teriyaki Ginger tuna Skewers	Goat cheese salad with slices of bacon and almonds	Carrot Ginger Soup and Cabbage Noodles
	Celery sticks and almond butter	Bell Pepper Nachos	
Day 2	Volcano eggs	Cheeseburger Soup	Pecan crusted salmon
	Cheddar Taco Crisps	Crab and Avocado duet	
Day 3	Avocado smoothie	Duck barbecue with grilled zucchini and eggplants	Turkey Involtini
	Apple with almond butter	Celery sticks and almond butter	
Day 4	Cheesy veggie omelet	Mongolian Beef	Cauliflower mac and cheese
	Cheesy Cauliflower Breadsticks	Roast beef and sliced cheese	
Day 5	Zucchini bread	Instant Pot Crack Chicken	Pork chop with cabbage slaw
	Kale chips	Crab and Avocado duet	
Day 6	Raspberry Chia Jars	Flaxseed crusted chicken tenders	Meatballs and Zucchini noodles
	Bell Pepper Nachos	Sugar-free turkey jerky	
Day 7	Fried eggs, bacon, and green salad	Chicken Pizza	Potato Salad
	Celery sticks and almond butter	Citrus marinated olives	

Cook Healthy, Eat Healthily

Here's another modified meal plan made for week three. Remember that you can follow or change this plan according to how you intend to use it. The meals listed below are lifted from the sample recipes included in this guide. The purpose of creating a meal plan is to help you to watch what you are about to consume and make sure you're meeting your daily nutrition needs.

Week 3 Modified Keto Diet Sample Meal Plan

	AM (breakfast and snack)	Noon (lunch and snack)	PM (dinner and snack)
Day 1	Macadamia bread	Tuna salad with romaine lettuce	Baked tofu with Cauliflower rice
	Kale chips	Cheddar Taco Crisps	
Day 2	Chia seed pudding	Pork Rolls with Provolone cheese	White Chicken Chili
	Roast beef and sliced cheese	Sugar-free turkey jerky	
Day 3	Broccoli Cheese Bites	Spinach salad	Roast Beef and cheese
	Celery sticks and almond butter	Almonds	

Day			
Day 4	Breakfast sandwiches	Egg Salad	Cauliflower pizza with mozzarella
	Cheesy Cauliflower Breadsticks	Bacon-wrapped shrimp and scallops	
Day 5	Baked eggs in avocado cups	Garlic Butter Pork Chops	Grilled shrimp topped with lemon
	Citrus marinated olives	Bell Pepper Nachos	
Day 6	Tuna Salad cups	Sashimi and miso soup	Ground Beef Casserole
	Apple with almond butter	Roast beef and sliced cheese	
Day 7	Keto Cinnamon Rolls	Salmon Patties	Stuffed Pork Roast
	Sugar-free turkey jerky	Cheddar Taco Crisps	

SAMPLE RECIPES

Roasted Veggies

Ingredients:

- 1/2 lb. turnips
- 1/2 lb. carrots
- 1/2 lb. parsnips
- 2 shallots, peeled
- 1/4 tsp. ground black pepper
- 1 tbsp. extra-virgin olive oil
- 6 cloves garlic
- 3/4 tsp. kosher salt
- 2 tbsp. fresh rosemary needles

Instructions:

1. First, cut vegetables into bite-sized pieces.
2. Set the oven to 400°F.
3. Mix all the ingredients in a baking dish.
4. Roast the vegetables for 25 minutes until brown and tender.
5. Toss and roast again for 20–25 minutes.
6. Serve and enjoy while hot.

Spinach and Watercress Salad

Ingredients:

- 1 cup watercress, washed with stems removed
- 3 cups baby spinach, washed with stems removed
- 1 medium sliced avocado
- 1/4 cup avocado oil
- 1/8 cup lemon juice
- a pinch of salt

Instructions:

1. Pat dry the spinach and watercress. Remove the stem and separate the leaves.
2. On a large serving plate, combine the leaves of the watercress and the spinach.
3. Cut the avocado in half, then remove the pit. Peel the skin off from each side.
4. Slice the avocados into thin strips. Set aside.
5. Prepare the dressing by combining avocado oil and lemon juice.
6. Arrange the avocado strips on top of the watercress and spinach.
7. Season with salt and pepper.
8. Drizzle with the dressing before serving.

Keto Pesto Chicken

Ingredients:

- 1-1/2 lbs chicken thighs breasts, boneless and cut into bite-sized pieces
- pepper
- salt
- 2 tbsp. butter or coconut oil
- 5 tbsp. red or green pesto
- 1-1/4 cups heavy whipping cream
- 5 oz. feta cheese, diced
- 3 oz. pitted olives
- 1 garlic clove, finely chopped

Salad:

- 5 oz. leafy greens
- 4 tbsp. olive oil
- sea salt
- ground black pepper

Instructions:

1. Preheat the oven to 400°F.
2. Season the chicken with salt and pepper.
3. Add butter or oil to a large skillet. Fry the chicken pieces on medium-high heat until golden brown.
4. In a bowl, combine heavy cream and pesto. Mix well.
5. Put the fried chicken meat in a baking dish. Add in olives, garlic, and feta cheese.

6. Pour the pesto or cream mixture.
7. Bake in the oven for 20-30 minutes.
8. Toss all the salad ingredients upon serving.
9. Serve and enjoy.

Mixed Vegetable Roast with Lemon Zest

Ingredients:

- 1-1/2 cups broccoli florets
- 1-1/2 cups cauliflower florets
- 3/4 cup red bell pepper, diced
- 3/4 cup zucchini, diced
- 2 thinly sliced cloves of garlic
- 2 tsp. lemon zest
- 1 tbsp. olive oil
- a pinch of salt
- 1 tsp. dried and crushed oregano

Instructions:

1. Preheat the oven to 425°F for 25 minutes.
2. Combine garlic and florets of broccoli and cauliflower in a baking pan.
3. Drizzle oil evenly over the vegetables. Season with salt and oregano.
4. Stir the vegetables to coat them evenly.
5. Place the pan inside the oven and roast for 10 minutes.

6. Add zucchini and bell pepper to the mix. Toss to combine.
7. Continue roasting for 10 to 15 minutes more until the vegetables turn light brown.
8. Drizzle lemon zest over vegetables and toss.
9. Serve and enjoy.

Salmon and Asparagus

Ingredients:

- 2 salmon filets
- 14-oz. young potatoes
- 8 asparagus spears, trimmed and halved
- 2 handfuls cherry tomatoes
- 1 handful basil leaves
- 2 tbsp. extra-virgin olive oil
- 1 tbsp. balsamic vinegar

Instructions:

1. Heat oven to 428°F.
2. Arrange potatoes into a baking dish.
3. Drizzle potatoes with extra-virgin olive oil.
4. Roast potatoes until they have turned golden brown.
5. Place asparagus into the baking dish together with the potatoes.
6. Roast in the oven for 15 minutes.
7. Arrange cherry tomatoes and salmon among the vegetables.

8. Drizzle with balsamic vinegar and the remaining olive oil.
9. Roast until the salmon is cooked.
10. Throw in basil leaves before transferring everything to a serving dish.
11. Serve while hot.

Arugula and Mushroom Salad

Ingredients:

- 5 oz. arugula washed
- 1 lb. fresh mushrooms
- 1/4 tsp. shoyu
- 1/2 red onion
- 1 tbsp. olive oil
- 1 tbsp. mirin

For tofu cheese:

- 1/8 cup umeboshi vinegar
- 1/2 firm tofu

Instructions:

1. In a bowl, add the rinsed tofu. Crumble and pour in vinegar.
2. In a separate bowl add shoyu, red onions, salt, olive oil, and mirin. 3. Mix to combine.
3. Add in the arugula and toss to combine with the dressing.

4. Serve and enjoy.

Seafood Stew

Ingredients:

- 2 tsp. extra-virgin olive oil
- 1 cut bulb fennel
- 2 stalks celery, chopped
- 2 cups white wine
- 1 tbsp. chopped thyme
- 1 cup chopped shallots
- 6 ounces shrimp
- 6 ounces of sea scallops
- 1/4 tsp. salt
- 1 cup chopped parsley
- 6 oz. Arctic char
- 2-1/2 cups of water

Instructions:

1. Heat a frying pan on the lowest setting. Add a small amount of oil.
2. Cook the celery, shallots, and fennel for approximately 6 minutes.
3. Pour the wine, water, and thyme into the frying pan.
4. Wait for 10 minutes and allow it to cook.
5. Once much of the water has evaporated, add in the remaining ingredients, and wait for 2 minutes before removing it from the stove.
6. Serve and enjoy immediately.

Keto Taco Shells

Ingredients:

- 60 grams of fresh spinach leaves
- 2 eggs
- 1/3 cup almond meal
- 2 tsp psyllium husk
- 1/2 tsp salt
- taco toppings
- smoked chicken
- avocado
- onion
- sour cream
- tomato
- coriander
- chipotle adobo sauce or any low carb sauce

Instruction:

1. Preheat the oven to 160-180°C.
2. Prepare a pan lined with baking paper.
3. Pour the spinach leaves over boiling water and cover for 5 minutes to blanch.
4. Drain and squeeze afterward.
5. Put the spinach into a food processor together with eggs, psyllium husk, and almond meal, then season with salt. Process until fine and smooth.

6. Make 15 cm big circles by placing approximately a quarter of the mixture onto the pan and spreading it by using a cranked spatula.
7. Afterward, place in the oven and bake for about 9 minutes or until cooked.
8. Set aside to cool and then bake again for another 10 minutes to dry.
9. Once done, fill it with taco toppings and serve.

Tomato Clams

Ingredients:

- Canola oil cooking spray
- 1 onion, sliced
- 1 tsp. minced garlic, or to taste
- 1/2 tsp salt
- 3 pounds of clams, in shell, thoroughly scrubbed
- 1 tsp red pepper flakes
- 1 cup white wine
- 1/2 lb. whole-grain linguine, cooked according to package directions
- 1/2 cup flat-leaf parsley, chopped
- 4 cups cherry tomatoes, halved

Instructions:

1. Heat a large pot with a lid over low heat.
2. Spray with vegetable oil cooking spray and add the onion, garlic, and salt. Cook for 3 minutes, stirring constantly.

3. Add the clams, red pepper flakes, and wine
4. Cover and simmer until the clams open, approximately 7 minutes. Discard those clams that do not open.
5. Add the pasta, parsley, and tomatoes.
6. Cover and let simmer for an additional 3 minutes.
7. Stir and serve immediately.

Chicken Soup

Ingredients:

- 4 cups low-sodium, fat-free chicken broth
- 2 cups skinless and organic chicken, boiled and diced
- 2 carrots, diced
- 1 red onion, chopped
- 3/4 cup turnip, diced
- 1/2 cup fresh parsley, chopped

Instructions:

1. Using medium heat, boil the chicken broth in a large saucepan.
2. Add the carrots, onion, turnip, and parsley to the broth.
3. Reduce the heat from medium to low. Cover the saucepan.
4. Simmer until the vegetables are tender.
5. Add the diced chicken.
6. Simmer the soup for another 3 to 4 minutes.
7. Serve and enjoy while hot.

Keto Zucchini Walnut Bread

Ingredients:

- 3 large eggs
- 1/2 cup virgin olive oil
- 1 tsp. vanilla extract
- 2-1/4 cups fine almond flour
- 1-1/2 cups sweetener, erythritol
- 1/2 tsp. salt
- 1-1/2 tsp. baking powder
- 1/2 tsp. nutmeg, ground
- 1 tsp. cinnamon, ground
- 1/4 tsp. ginger, ground
- 1 cup zucchini, grated
- 1/2 cup walnuts, chopped

Instructions:

1. Preheat your oven to 350°F.
2. Whisk together the eggs, oil, and vanilla extract. Set aside.
3. Using another bowl, combine the baking powder, sweetener, almond flour, salt, cinnamon, nutmeg, and ginger powder. Set aside.
4. Squeeze the excess water from the zucchini using a paper towel or a cheesecloth.
5. Pour the zucchini into the egg mixture and whisk.
6. Add the flour mixture slowly into the egg and zucchini mixture. Blend using an electric blender until the mixture turns smooth.

7. Spray a loaf pan with avocado oil or baking spray.
8. Pour the zucchini batter into the loaf pan and smoothen the top evenly.
9. Spoon the chopped walnuts on top of the batter, lightly pressing the walnuts with the back of a spoon to press into the batter.
10. Pop the loaf pan into the oven and then bake for 60-70 minutes, or until the walnuts turn brown.
11. Cool in a cooling rack before slicing and serving.

Vegan Pesto

Ingredients:

- 1/3 cup olive oil (or other high-quality and flavorful oil)
- 1-1/2 cups basil, fresh
- 5 cloves garlic
- 1 cup pine nuts
- 1/3 cup nutritional yeast
- 3/4 tsp. salt
- 1/2 tsp. black pepper

Instructions:

1. In a food processor, add all the ingredients.
2. Start processing until the nuts are ground.
3. Add more salt and pepper to taste.

Spinach and Chickpeas

Ingredients:

- 3 tbsp. extra virgin olive oil
- 1 onion, thinly sliced
- 4 cloves garlic, minced
- 1 tbsp. grated ginger
- 1/2 container grape tomatoes
- 1 lemon, zested and freshly juiced
- 1 tsp. crushed red pepper flakes
- 1 large can of chickpeas
- 6 cups spinach
- sea salt

Instructions:

1. Add extra virgin olive oil to a large skillet, add onion, and cook until the onion starts to brown.
2. Add all the ingredients except for the chickpeas. Cook for 3 to 4 minutes.
3. Add cooked chickpeas and stir. Add oil if necessary.
4. Serve and enjoy.

Zucchini and Celery Greens Soup

Ingredients:

- 1/2 cup cooked green lentils
- 1 onion, finely diced

* 1 parsnip, peeled and finely diced
* 2 garlic cloves, crushed
* 1 green bell pepper, cut into small cubes
* 1 zucchini, sliced
* 4 asparagus spears
* 1 fennel bulb, diced finely
* 2 celery stalks, diced finely
* 1 small bunch of celery greens or other greens available: beet greens, kale, or spinach
* 2 cups low sodium vegetable broth
* 1 lime, juice only
* 1 tsp. chia seeds to garnish
* freshly ground black pepper

Instructions:

1. Stir-fry onion and garlic, for about 2 minutes.
2. Throw in the parsnip, bell pepper, fennel, celery stalks, and zucchini, along with the vegetable broth.
3. Wait until it boils. Then, lower the heat and let it simmer for 7 minutes.
4. Put in the asparagus, lime juice, lentils, and celery greens. Turn off the heat.
5. Serve warm, garnished with chia seeds.

Zero Carb Bread

Ingredients:

* 3 eggs

- 3 tbsp. cream cheese at room temperature
- 1/4 tsp. baking powder

Instructions:

1. Preheat the oven to 300°F.
2. Separate the yolk from the egg whites.
3. In one bowl, mix the egg yolks, cream cheese, and honey until smooth.
4. In a second bowl, add baking powder to the whites. Beat the whites with the hand mixer at high speed until they are fluffy.
5. Gently fold the egg yolk mixture into the egg white mixture.
6. Continue folding gently but swiftly to avoid melting the mixture. Make sure to not break the egg whites' fluffiness.
7. Spoon about 10-12 rounds of the mixture onto a lightly greased baking sheet.
8. Bake for 18-20 minutes on the middle rack.
9. Broil for a minute or a minute and a half, cooking the top until they become nice and golden brown.

Tahini Salmon

Instructions:

- 1/4 cup tahini
- 3 tbsp. fresh lemon juice
- 1 tsp. mashed garlic
- 1/4 tsp. salt

- 1/2 cup finely chopped cilantro
- 2 tbsp. roughly chopped toasted walnuts
- 2 tbsp. roughly chopped toasted almonds
- 1 tbsp. finely chopped onion
- 1 tsp. extra-virgin olive oil
- cayenne
- black pepper, freshly ground
- 1 lb. wild salmon skin removed, fresh or frozen

Instructions:

1. In a bowl, combine the tahini, 2 tbsp. of lemon juice, 3 tbsp. of water, mashed garlic, and 1/8 tsp. of salt; set aside
2. In a separate bowl, combine the cilantro, walnuts, almonds, onion, olive oil, cayenne, black pepper, and 1/8 tsp. of salt.
3. Fill the bottom of a steamer with water and bring it to a boil.
4. Season fish with 1 tbsp. of lemon juice.
5. Place it on a plate and put it on top of the steamer. Cover and cook, taking care to remove while the fish is still pink inside, about 3 to 4 minutes.
6. Remove the fish from the steamer, top with the tahini mixture, and then with the cilantro mixture.
7. Serve warm or at room temperature.

Tomato and Basil Soup

Ingredients:

- 1 medium-sized onion, chopped
- 1 clove garlic, sliced finely
- 2 tablespoons olive oil
- 3 pcs. vine tomatoes or 8 pcs. cherry tomatoes, chopped
- 400 g can plum tomatoes
- 150 ml water
- 5 leaves of fresh basil or 1 tsp. dried basil
- 1 tsp. salt
- pepper

Instructions:

1. Sauté onion, tomatoes, garlic, and basil in olive oil.
2. Pour in the canned tomatoes. Add salt and pepper.
3. Cover and let it simmer for 30 minutes on low heat.
4. Transfer to a blender or food processor and blend until smooth.
5. Serve and enjoy.

Cauliflower and Mushroom Bake

Ingredients:

- 3 cups cauliflower florets
- 1 cup fresh mushroom, chopped
- 1/2 cup red onion, chopped
- 1/3 cup green onion, chopped
- 2 garlic cloves, finely chopped
- 2 tsp. apple cider vinegar

- 2 tsp. lemon juice
- 1/2 tsp. salt
- 1/4 tsp. pepper*
- 1 tbsp. olive oil

Instructions:

1. Preheat the oven to 350°F. Lightly grease a baking pan.
2. Combine red onion, cauliflower, olive oil, garlic, mushroom, apple cider vinegar, lemon juice, salt, and pepper in a bowl. Mix well.
3. Pour the mixture into the greased baking pan.
4. Place inside the oven and bake for 45 minutes. Stir.
5. When vegetables are golden brown and tender, remove them from the oven.
6. Garnish with green onions. Serve and enjoy.

***black pepper may be substituted with white pepper**

Ketogenic Pizza

Ingredients:

Crust:

- 4 eggs
- 6 oz. shredded cheese, mozzarella or provolone

Toppings:

- 1 tsp. dried oregano

* 3 tbsp. unsweetened tomato sauce
* 1-1/2 oz. pepperoni
* 5 oz. shredded cheese
* optional: olives optional

Salad:

* 4 tbsp. olive oil
* 2 oz. leafy greens
* ground black pepper
* sea salt

Instructions:

1. Prepare the oven by preheating to 400°F.
2. Stir eggs and shredded cheese into a medium-sized bowl.
3. Transfer the batter on a baking sheet with parchment paper.
4. Bake until the crust turns golden, about 15 minutes.
5. Once done, take it out and leave to cool for 1-2 minutes.
6. Adjust the temperature of the oven to about 450°F.
7. On the crust, put tomato sauce and sprinkle oregano.
8. Add cheese, followed by pepperoni and olives.
9. Bake in the oven for about 5-10 minutes.
10. Toss the ingredients of the salad.
11. Serve immediately.

Cajun-Style Chicken Wrap

Ingredients:

- 1 large whole wheat keto tortilla
- 1/2 avocado, chopped
- 4 oz. cajun chicken, breast part, chopped and cooked
- 1/2 beefsteak tomato, chopped
- 2 tbsp. yogurt, preferably plain or organic
- 1-1/2 cups lettuce, chopped
- 1/3 cup cucumber, chopped
- pepper, to taste
- sea salt, to taste

Instructions:

1. Except for the tortilla, toss all the ingredients for the salad in a bowl.
2. Heat up the tortilla in the microwave for 15 seconds, then plate it nicely.
3. Gently transfer the salad mix to the center of the tortilla. Once done, fold both sides nicely, similar to how a burrito is wrapped.
4. Slice and enjoy eating.

Egg Roll Bowl

Ingredients:

- 1 package of defrosted egg roll wrappers, cut into 0.5x3-inch per piece
- 1.5 lbs. ground pork
- 3 small cloves of garlic, minced
- 2 tsp. fresh ginger, peeled and minced

- 1/2 cup vegetable or chicken broth
- 1/3 cup coconut aminos
- 1.5 tsp. toasted sesame oil
- 1 9-oz. package pre-shredded cabbage
- 3-4 green onions, chopped
- sriracha sauce

Instructions:

1. Preheat the oven to 400°F.
2. Place wrappers on a baking sheet. Brush with a little olive oil.
3. Bake for about 5 minutes, or until golden brown.
4. In a large pan, heat 1 tbsp. of oil over medium-high heat.
5. Add raw meat. Cook for about 4-5 minutes, or until golden brown.
6. Drain or pat with a paper towel after removing from the pan.
7. Raw meat is browned in a pan
8. In the same pan, turn the heat to medium. Add garlic and ginger, and stir occasionally for about a minute.
9. Add cabbage slaw mix and most of the green onions. Cook for around 3 minutes until softened.
10. Add broth, coconut amino, and sesame oil. Stir well.
11. Scoop up the ingredients into a bowl.
12. Top with toasted egg roll wrappers, sriracha, and leftover green onions.

Mushroom Omelet

Ingredients:

- 3 eggs
- 1 oz. butter, for frying
- 1 oz. shredded cheese
- 1/4 yellow onion, chopped
- 4 large mushrooms, sliced
- salt
- pepper

Instructions:

1. Whisk eggs with a pinch of salt and pepper until smooth.
2. Melt the butter in a frying pan, over medium heat.
3. Toss in mushrooms and onions. Stir until tender.
4. Pour in the egg mixture, covering the bottom of the pan.
5. Before the omelet completely sets on top, sprinkle cheese.
6. Fold over the omelet in half.
7. Serve and enjoy.

Conclusion

Thank you again for getting this guide.

If you found this guide helpful, please take the time to share your thoughts and post a review. It'd be greatly appreciated!

Thank you and good luck!

References and Helpful Links

Are you missing nutrients on a low-carb diet? (n.d.). Verywell Fit. Retrieved April 1, 2023, from https://www.verywellfit.com/low-carb-diet-nutrient-deficiencies-2242236.

Cipryan, L., Plews, D. J., Ferretti, A., Maffetone, P. B., & Laursen, P. B. (2018). Effects of a 4-week very low-carbohydrate diet on high-intensity interval training responses. Journal of Sports Science & Medicine, 17(2), 259–268. https://www.ncbi.nlm.nih.gov/pmc/articles/PMC5950743/.

Keto 2. 0 is here to make the low-carb diet way better for you—And easier to follow. (2019, December 11). Prevention. https://www.prevention.com/weight-loss/diets/a30196446/keto-2-0-diet/.

Macronutrients | national agricultural library. (n.d.). Retrieved April 1, 2023, from https://www.nal.usda.gov/human-nutrition-and-food-safety/food-composition/macronutrients.

Medicine, C. for F. (2019, March 13). 4 vitamin deficiencies found in low carb diets. Center for Family Medicine - Sherman Texas. https://centerforfamilymedicine.com/nutritional-information/4-vitamin-deficiencies-found-in-low-carb-diets/.

Should you try the keto diet? 2023 Beginner's Guide | Best Diets. (n.d.). Retrieved April 1, 2023, from https://health.usnews.com/best-diet/keto-diet.

The keto diet is super hard—These 3 variations are much easier to follow. (n.d.). Health. Retrieved April 1, 2023, from https://www.health.com/weight-loss/keto-diet-types.

What is the modified keto diet? - Perfect keto. (n.d.). Retrieved April 1, 2023, from https://perfectketo.com/modified-keto-diet/.

WHO EMRO | Double burden of nutrition | Nutrition site. (n.d.). World Health Organization - Regional Office for the Eastern Mediterranean. Retrieved April 1, 2023, from http://www.emro.who.int/nutrition/double-burden-of-nutrition/index.html.